GOPex

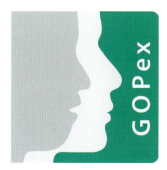

Performance Enhanced Growth!

www.forwardontics.com

GOPex
Good Oral Posture Exercises

© Second English Edition, 2019
ISBN: 978-0-9963349-6-9

Acknowledgments

To Dr. John Mew in recognition to his great service to humanity, to David, Ilan, and Ariela, for their patience and support.
Dr. Sandra Kahn

To Jeannie for believing, my Grandmother for remembering the old ways and John for unwavering in seeking truth.
Dr. Simon Wong

Texts: Dr. Sandra Kahn, Dr. Simon Wong
Graphic Design: Susan Szecsi
Illustrations: Susan Szecsi, Laura Liberatore, Dr. Sandra Kahn

GOPex
GOOD ORAL POSTURE EXERCISES

"Why on Earth are Orthodontists Talking About Posture?"

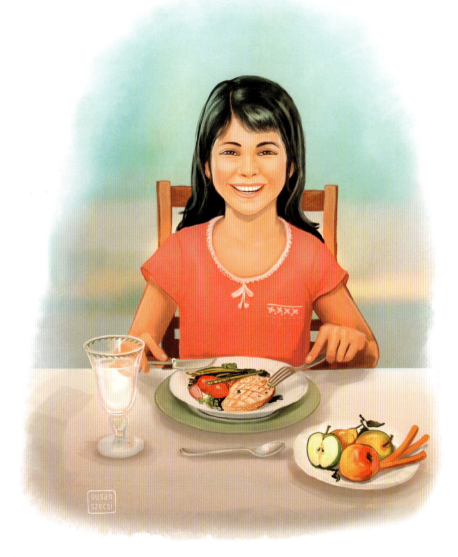

Actually, it's because we live on Earth. Here, your posture is very important. The "stance" and "mindset" you adopt, makes you who you are! This is your secret guide to being healthier, growing stronger and having straighter teeth!

TROPIC PREMISE

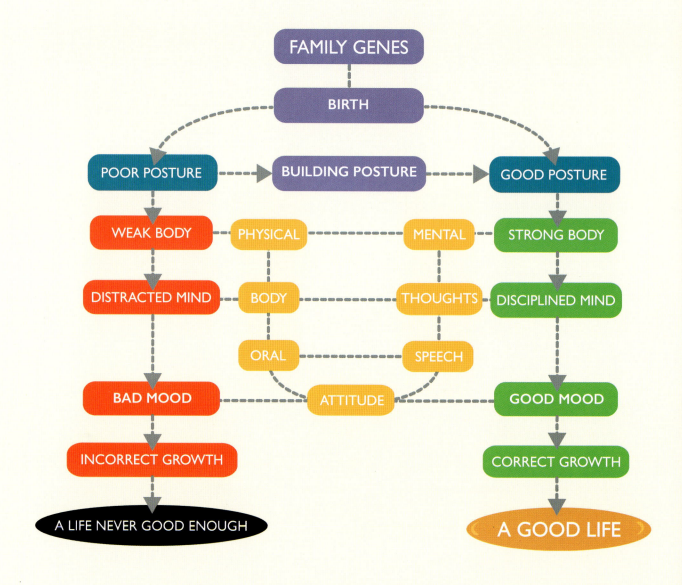

Your conditioning, or lack of it, has a huge impact on your growth and development. Good training will always result in correct growth. That is the "Tropic Premise".

INTRODUCTION

A book that will unite parents and children in their quest for a healthier and harmonious development.

This book was designed to help you develop correct resting oral posture. With it, you will achieve balanced growth of your face and teeth. Additionally, these exercises will support you in quest to develop your mind and body in the best way, so that you can reach your potential!

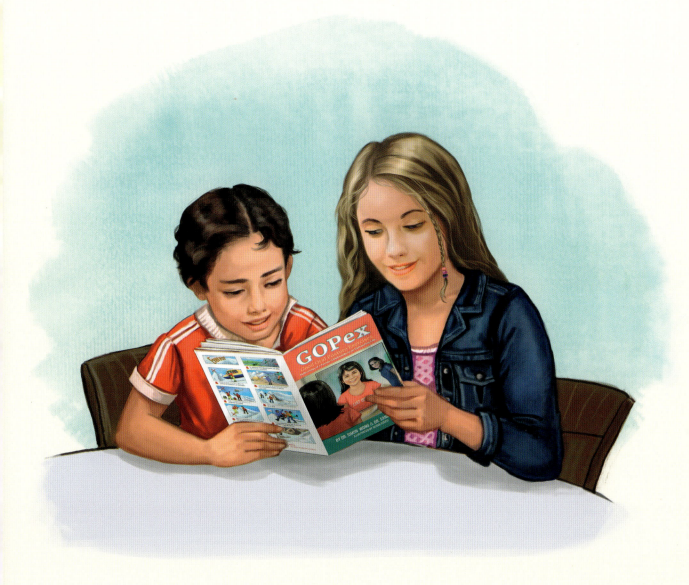

The "Why" and "What" of Correct Oral Posture

"The ideal development of the jaw and teeth is dependent on correct oral posture with the tongue resting on the palate, the lips sealed and the teeth in light contact between four and eight hours a day.[1]"

Your bones and teeth grow and move in response to the pressure of your muscles and skin. Maintaining your mouth fully closed at night during your sleep, "squeezes" out the most perfect version of you!

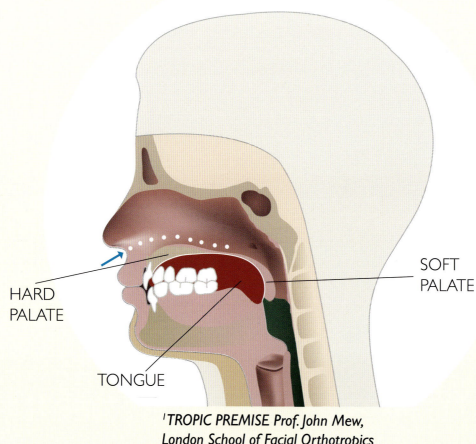

[1] TROPIC PREMISE Prof. John Mew,
London School of Facial Orthotropics

This book contains exercises that will help you naturally keep your mouth fully closed when you are at rest. After some time, you will do it without even thinking about it!

TROPIC PREMISE

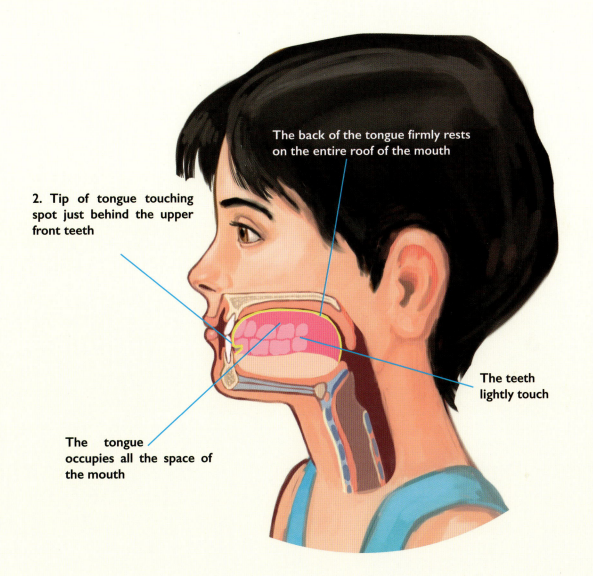

The back of the tongue firmly rests on the entire roof of the mouth

2. Tip of tongue touching spot just behind the upper front teeth

The teeth lightly touch

The tongue occupies all the space of the mouth

Correct oral posture means that the mouth is fully closed. That everything is touching – connected – harmoniously with no airspaces anywhere! When everything is tightly connected, your body naturally puts all the pieces together to match each one in the best way. Meaning that every part is going to grow in unity!

Nature requires proper posture for good growth and development.*

Before you are born, while you are developing, your mother protects you by keeping you safe in her body. As soon as you are born, all that changes. In order to survive, others must teach you how to be strong.
Look at the lady nursing her baby. Note her straight back, toned yet relaxed at the same time. Notice how she encourages proper development of her baby's hips and back by nursing her child at a natural angle. Nature requires proper posture for good growth and development.*

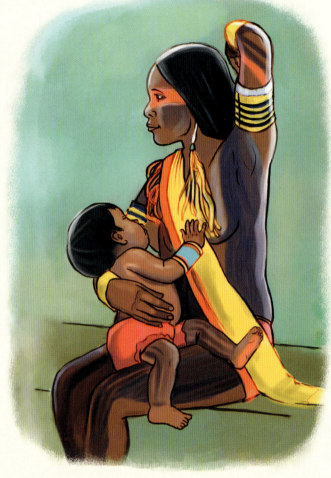

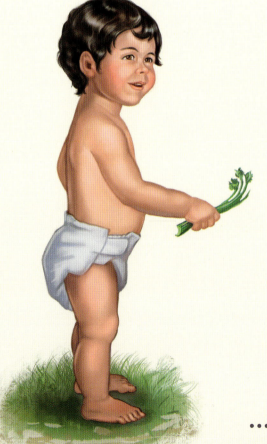

Look at the baby now.
Her hips are rotated forward. What can you tell us about her posture? Notice how the head is aligned with the neck and back – all straight.

Based on research of the ancient posture of "Eight steps to a pain-free back" Esther Gokhale.

In ancient times, children grew up strong, but now, modern life forces people to separate from what once was natural.

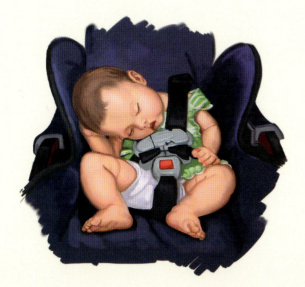

Look at the baby sitting on the car seat, not being held by his mother but by an object. What can you tell me about his position? How does it compare to the breastfed baby in her mother's arms? How does it compare to the baby on the opposite page?

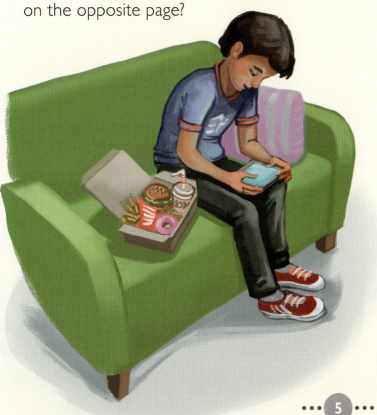

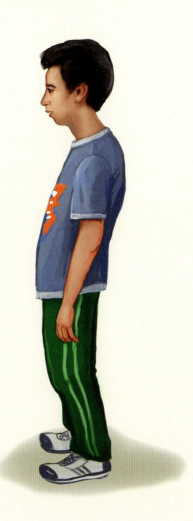

Is this slouching boy adopting a good posture?

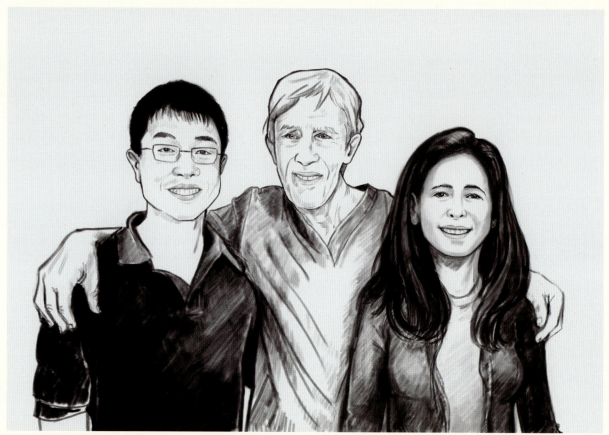

Dr. Simon Wong, Dr. John Mew and Dr. Sandra Kahn

The good news is that you can reverse the damage and return to the upstanding posture you were born to have.

Getting back to your natural posture is easier than you think!
Through this program, you will rewire your brain to help your body get back to the good posture you deserve. You will be excited and amazed to watch as your face and teeth become more balanced and straighter!

Before beginning the exercise program, you must make sure you have good back posture when sitting or standing.

GOOD SITTING POSTURE CHECKLIST

- Crown of head uplifted, as if it were gently lifted by a helium balloon;
- Mouth completely shut;
- Shoulders rolled back;
- Belly tucked in, under ribcage;
- Hips forward and butt back;
- Hands relaxed on the top of your thighs;
- Knees bent about 90 degrees in a chair that fits you properly;
- Both feet apart on the ground, at the same distance as your shoulders.

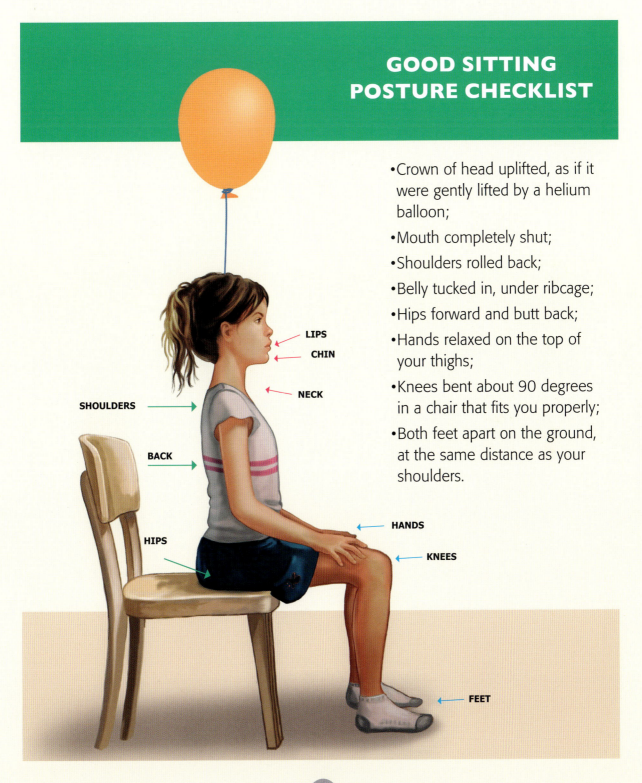

THE KEY TO GOOD POSTURE – STEP-BY-STEP

• **Feet**
Your feet must be well supported on the floor with even pressure ball to heel. If the chair is too high when sitting, you can use books or a stool so that your knees are around 90 degrees.
Have them both pointing forward and shoulder-width apart.

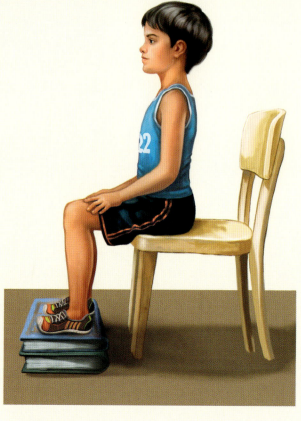

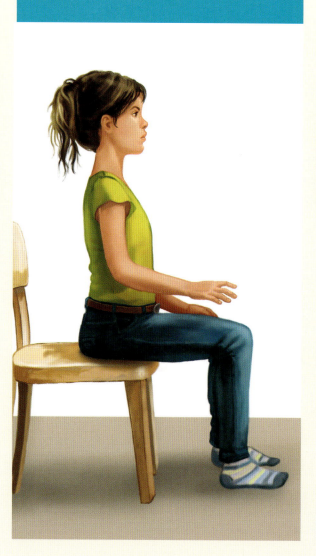

• **Hips**
The position of the hips when sitting or standing is of utmost importance when it comes to developing proper oral posture. As this will allow correct back posture and, hence, improved breathing. Imagine you are wearing a belt. Now, roll your hips until the buckle is lower than the belt hoop at the back.

• **Belly**
Tuck your belly in, imaging brushing it up under your rib cage.

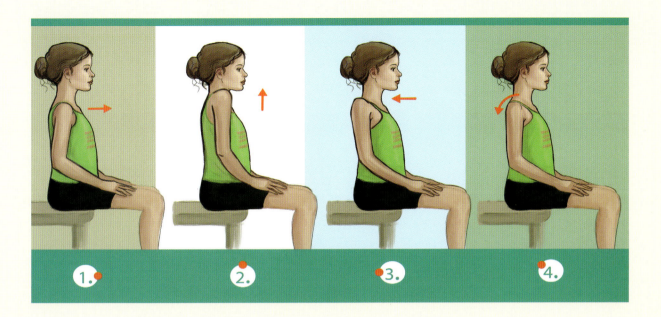

• **Shoulders**

To ensure that your shoulders are in the correct position, do shoulder rolls before starting; imagine that they are connected to a clock face.

1. Move your shoulders as far forward as you can;
2. Raise them as high as you can;
3. Then back, as far possible;
4. Now, relax them and let them fall gently, slightly behind the head and allow your hands to rest on your thighs, thumbs on top, fingers to the side.

SEE HOW EASY?

Now that you know how to sit properly make sure you go through this checklist every time you sit. You will feel that you are full of energy and will look powerfully strong!

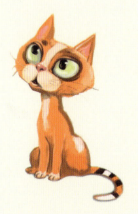

GOOD STANDING POSTURE CHECKLIST

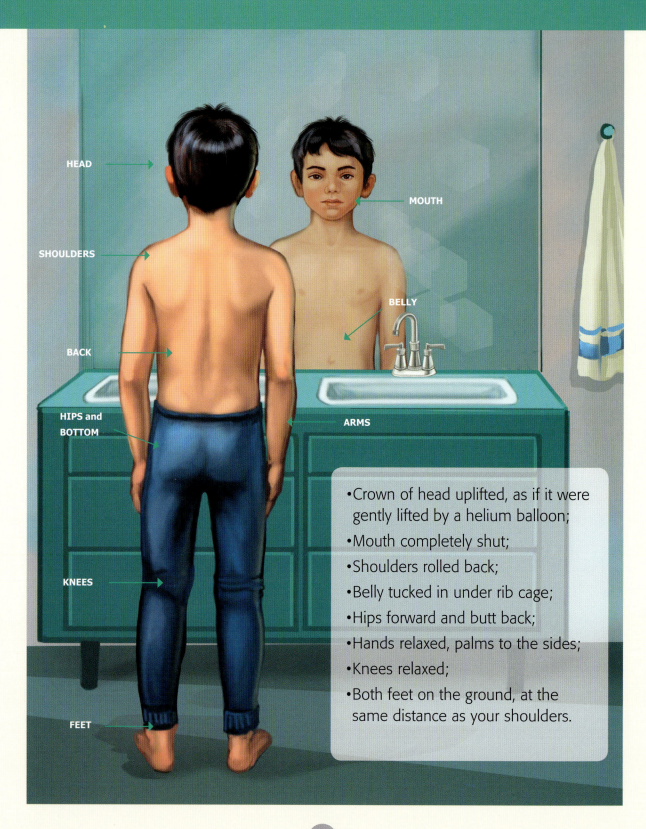

- Crown of head uplifted, as if it were gently lifted by a helium balloon;
- Mouth completely shut;
- Shoulders rolled back;
- Belly tucked in under rib cage;
- Hips forward and butt back;
- Hands relaxed, palms to the sides;
- Knees relaxed;
- Both feet on the ground, at the same distance as your shoulders.

DR. WONG'S GOPEX EXERCISES

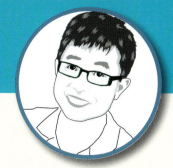

THE 4 CORNERSTONES TO HEALTH:

1) Resting with your mouth fully closed
2) Nose-only breathing at rest
3) Chewing hard (Like you mean it)
4) Swallowing softly (with your teeth together)

With this in mind, these exercises not only focus on improving how you rest but will also strengthen your jaw muscles. This will make you stronger and fitter.

FINDING CORRECT ORAL POSTURE

These two exercises will help you find the position for the tongue.

a) Letter "N" position

Pronounce "N" and then immediately shut your mouth with the lips together, teeth together, tongue and roof palate together. Feel your tongue tip on the "spot" just behind your front upper teeth and feel the back of your tongue high on the roof as well.

Keep your tongue stuck up like a planet sticker on your bedroom ceiling.

b) "Soft Swallow"

With you mouth closed, lips together, teeth together, tongue and roof palate together, gently lift your tongue even higher from front to back until you softly swallow.

Feel your tongue rise and throat fall but keep your teeth and lips soft, soft, soft together!

If you stay very, very soft when you finish your swallow, you will have quiet and lovely posture!!

FIND THE CORRECT ORAL POSTURE

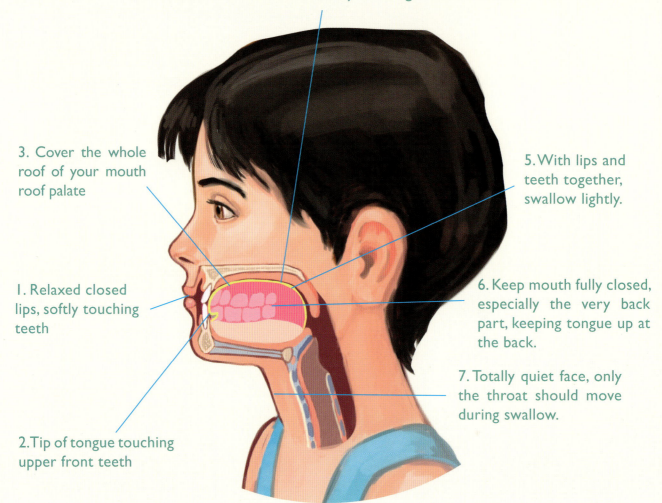

4. Seal whole roof of mouth with your tongue like a sticker

3. Cover the whole roof of your mouth roof palate

5. With lips and teeth together, swallow lightly.

1. Relaxed closed lips, softly touching teeth

6. Keep mouth fully closed, especially the very back part, keeping tongue up at the back.

7. Totally quiet face, only the throat should move during swallow.

2. Tip of tongue touching upper front teeth

Then with your teeth still together, softly lift your tongue high up until your swallow. You need to focus on keeping the muscles of your lips and face very still.

Lips together, teeth together, tongue in the roof of your mouth. Everything up, up, up but soft, soft, soft!

BUILDING GOOD MUSCLE TONE

With these exercises you will learn to rest correctly between chewing your food and building up your jaw muscles. Sit as we have shown you. Choose food that will strengthen your teeth and jaw, such as: lightly cooked vegetables, meat and whole fruits. No processed foods because they are designed to be soft – they are no challenge for your muscles and won't make you stronger!

CHEWING EXERCISE

Choose hard natural whole foods (not the soft processed factory foods, eww!). Take a bite and chew until it turns into mush (15-20 times). Keep your lips closed! Savor it for one second with the lips and teeth lightly touching. Remember, this part of the exercise is the important bit!!

Then, with your teeth still together, swallow. You need to focus on keeping the muscles of the outside of your face still.

Only movements on the inside!

Remember, always chew with your lips together and always swallow with all teeth touching.

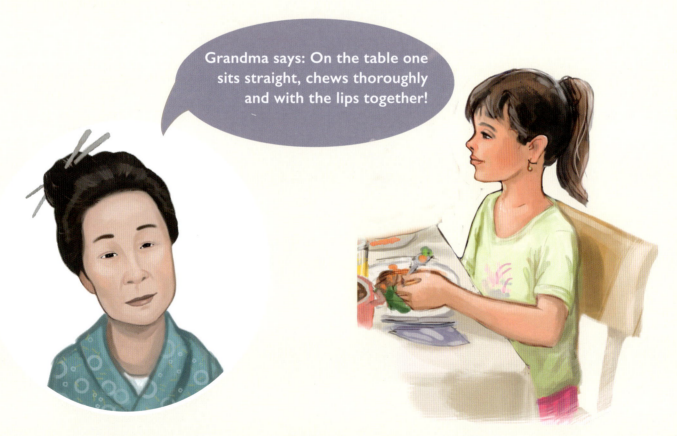

Grandma says: On the table one sits straight, chews thoroughly and with the lips together!

CHEWING EXERCISES BUILD GOOD MUSCLE TONE

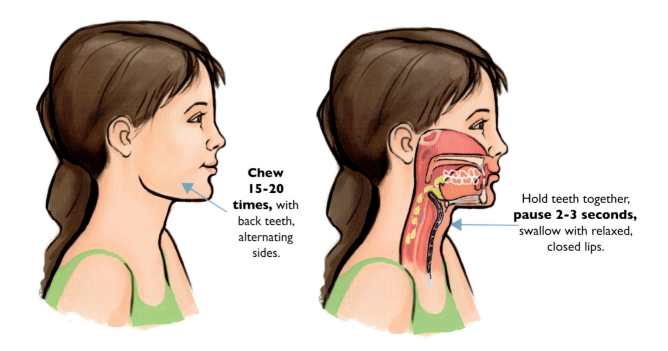

Chew 15-20 times, with back teeth, alternating sides.

Hold teeth together, **pause 2-3 seconds,** swallow with relaxed, closed lips.

BUSY IN THE INSIDE – QUIET ON THE OUTSIDE!

Practice these chewing exercises during the family meal time. At first, set aside some time every dinner to do this a couple of minutes. Then, later on, dedicate time to this every meal.
Remember, the only way to reach this goal is to chew like you mean it and swallow with your teeth together!

Repeat, repeat, repeat… and then you will start doing it, naturally, without even realizing!

Compare the poor posture of the child sitting on the right with the good posture of the girl sitting on the left. What are the differences you notice? Remember, the only way to reach your goal is to chew like you mean it!

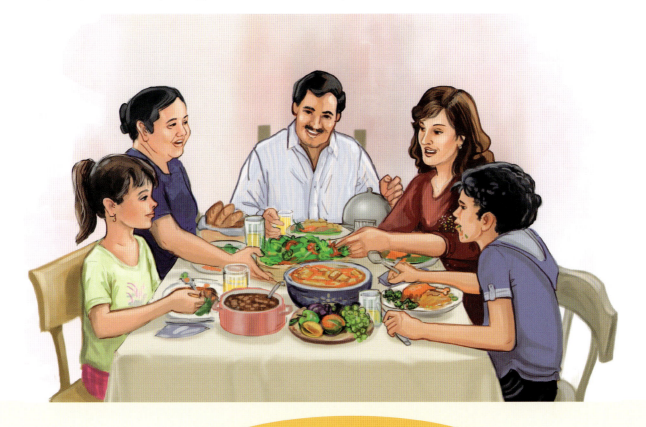

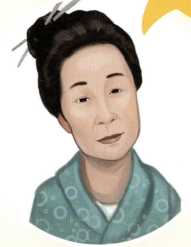

Do not distract yourself by reading, watching television, using computers or phones while you eat. You will not see fast results if you do not give these exercises 100% of your attention.

Developing nasal-only breathing teaches your brain that you need to rest with your mouth closed. This practice helps us maintain a closed mouth even when sleeping!

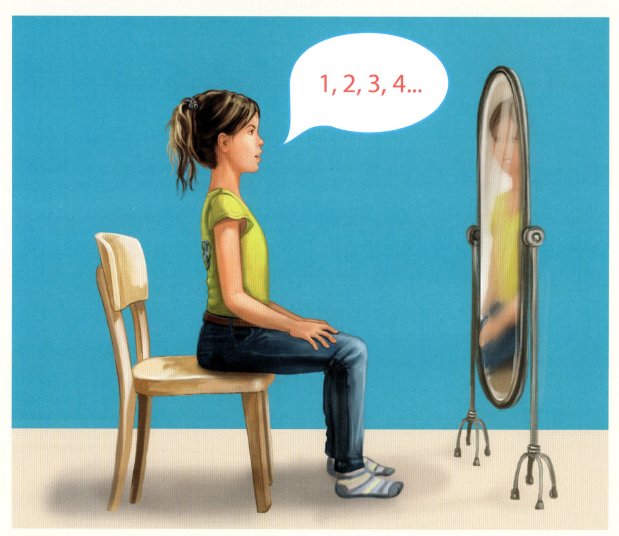

COUNTING EXERCISE

Slowly count out loud from 1 to 60 (or 30 for the very young). Pause to breathe through your nose at each count of 5. Aim to touch your teeth/lips between each count. Once in the morning and once in the evening please!

Remember, in the exercise, each time you pause, close your mouth and breathe only through your nose.

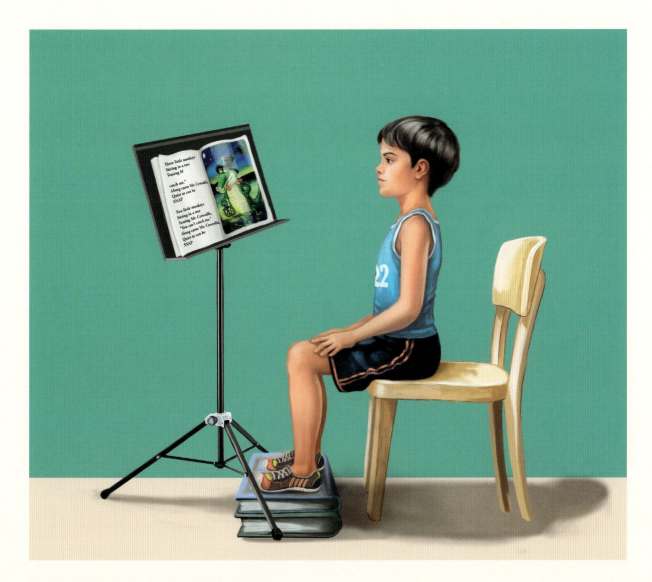

READING ALOUD EXERCISE

Reading aloud is an excellent practical application of this process. It only takes 5-20 minutes each day, reading out loud and punctuating each sentence correctly. With each comma and full stop, remember to pause with your mouth fully closed (in the "Click Click-Close" position!) and breathe in only through your nose.

Make sure to sit or stand with your back straight and your shoulders relaxed as we show on pages 7 and 9. Place the text you want to read on a music stand or a convenient place so you can keep the book at eye level. Imagine you are reading a paragraph in front of your school assembly. Speak slowly and clearly, pronouncing each word correctly. When you need to breathe, do so through your nose.

When you start these exercises you might feel like you are short of breath. This is normal. Keep at it with consistent practice, before long you'll be fit enough to breathe only through your nose with no difficulties.

To really make a difference and make these exercises change your posture, you must repeat and repeat them until your brain makes your body automatically close your mouth and keep it closed whenever you rest.

Do you know what type of punctuation allows you to breathe in through your mouth rather than only your nose when reading GOPEx style?

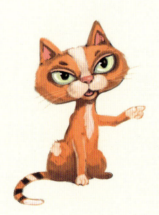

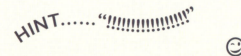

Exclamation marks (!) represent a peak in emotion. At these times it is correct to take breathe through your mouth, as you would naturally if you were shocked!

We recommend you take a simple challenge in order to convert simple changes into lifelong, positive habits. We ask you to do the exercises, every day, for 30 days in a row, without missing a single day!

We call this the 30-day challenge! Make sure everyone in your family helps you out, and show them that you can do it!

30-DAY CHALLENGE

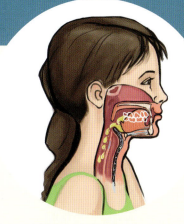

2 MINUTES OF CHEWING LIKE YOU MEAN IT

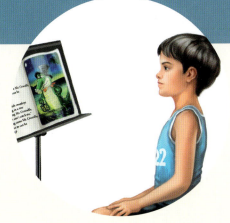

5 MINUTES OF READING ALOUD

Good oral posture will help you grow stronger, become fitter, sleep more peacefully and help you look smarter too! This is really important for your body and mind to be happy. For you to change, you have to convince your brain to take this seriously. Normally your brain is preoccupied with many things at once: with school, with friends, with what you're eating, with video games, with your pet's mischief, with a scrape on your knee, and other daily annoyances. That's why, unless your body gets used to doing the same thing all the time, it is very difficult to get your brain to pay attention to something in particular. Sometimes our brain behaves like a spoiled elf, that when something is difficult, it gives-in to laziness. What can you do to prevent this malicious elf from getting away with it? Here's the secret:

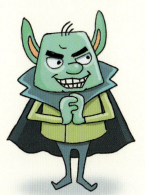

If you do something with complete conviction, seriousness and you are consistent - that is, no flops and no excuses - your brain will also take it seriously and help you do the exercises automatically, without you having to remember them! This is the kind of discipline you need to achieve all your goals!

Do something seriously enough times and it changes you! How much time you ask? Well 30 days in a row, should about do it! BUT you have to mean it for your brain to want to help you out, so **YOU CAN'T EVEN MISS ONE DAY IN THE THIRTY!**

Are You Brave Enough for this Challenge?

To make it simple you have to focus on the two most important exercises: chewing and reading.

For 30 DAYS IN A ROW devote two minutes to chewing and swallowing every meal as we show on page 14, and five to ten minutes to reading every night as we show on page 17.

Remember: YOU CAN'T MISS A SINGLE DAY. If you miss, even one day, you must start again from the beginning. In the table provided in this book, please mark your progress every day as you do the exercises. They only take about 10 minutes a day, so you have no excuses for not doing them daily!

To help you in your special mission, make sure your parents supervise you. You can even ask for our help. Have Mom or Dad use the app to videotape 30 seconds and send to a GOPex reviwer.

You will also have fun and learn a lot from watching your progress in the videos!

> Important!
> Remember you can only change if you take this seriously. Doing just some of the exercises for a limited time, simply tells your brain not to pay attention to it. If you really want to change your posture, by doing this daily you will show your brain how important this is. Show your brain who rules!

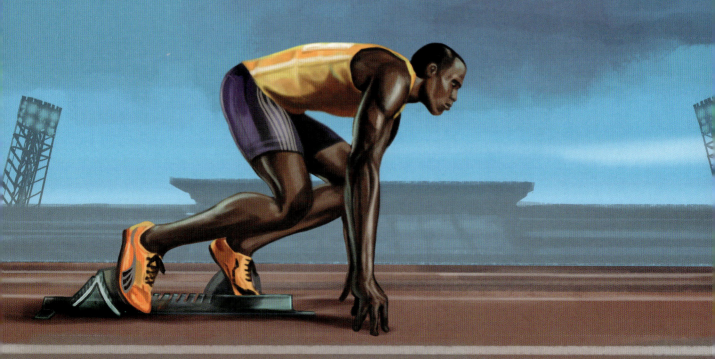

THE FINISHING EXERCISES TO IMPROVE REST ORAL POSTURE

LEARN TO SMILE WITH AN OPEN MOUTH.
A beautiful smile is wide, balanced and relaxed. Here's a great way to teach your face to do it perfectly!
Stand up straight in front of the mirror and smile, showing your teeth and making sure your smile is nicely even. Hold it for 3-4 seconds. Do this 10 times every day and share it with everyone!

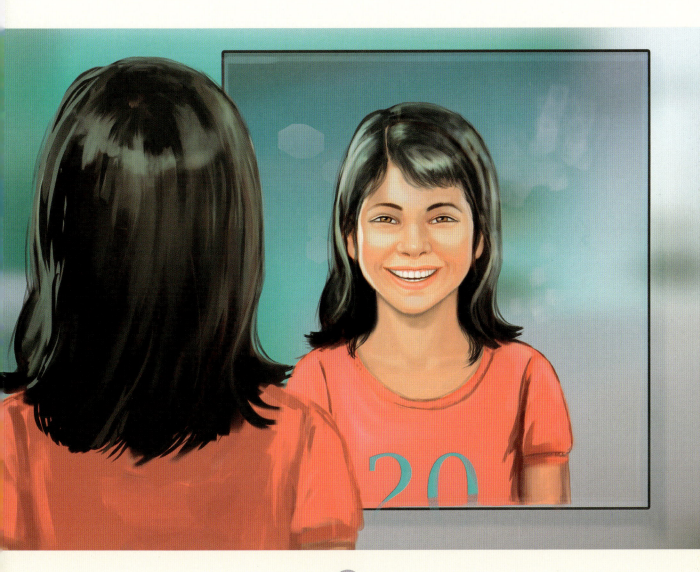

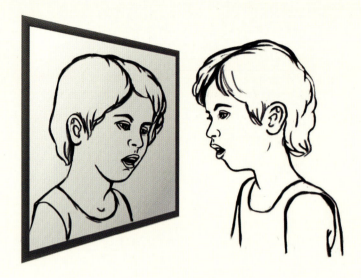

COMPARE YOUR POSTURE IN THE MIRROR

Stand in front of the mirror.
Try this, first stand slouching and with an open mouth. Consider how you look. Then, stand up straight and close your mouth fully. Note the difference.

Then, smile as you have practiced. Look at yourself. What do you think of yourself when you are like this?

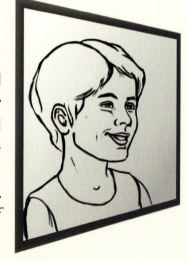 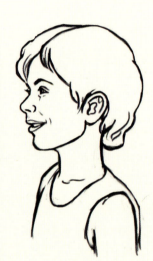

ALTITUDE AND ATTITUDE

We have had you focusing on your body posture.
The "altitude" is what puts you high up off the ground. But don't forget that posture also applies to your attitude or, in other words, "your mood".

Be committed and then do as you say you will. Keep your promises! Don't give Mom or Dad a hard time for reminding you of your chores and exercises.

If your parents forget to remind you to do your exercises, you remind them!

30-DAY CHALLENGE RESULTS

Once you've completed the **"30-day challenge"**, you will have established the commitment your brain needs to put your body to work and rest as nature intends.

YOU WILL BECOME STRONGER
It is hard work keeping your mouth closed. When you train your muscles to lift your jaw up all the time; that work pays off by building a stronger you!

YOU WILL DIGEST YOUR FOOD BETTER
Eating real food and mushing up the chunky bits for your stomach will make your body much happier!

YOU WILL SLEEP BETTER AND YOUR BODY WILL GROW STRAIGHTER
After you have programmed your brain to keep your mouth closed when you're at rest during the day, your brain will tell your body to sleep with your mouth closed too. This will allow more oxygen to fuel your body, as your nose filters, warms and moisturizes the air you breathe.

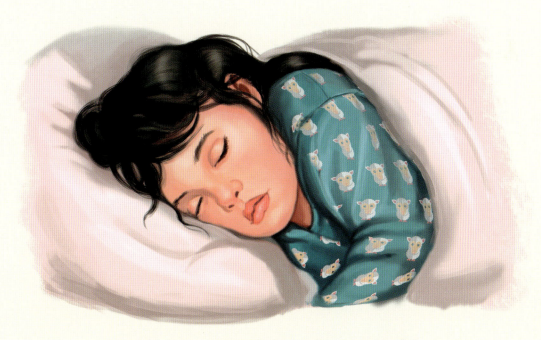

Nose breathing sleep is always peaceful

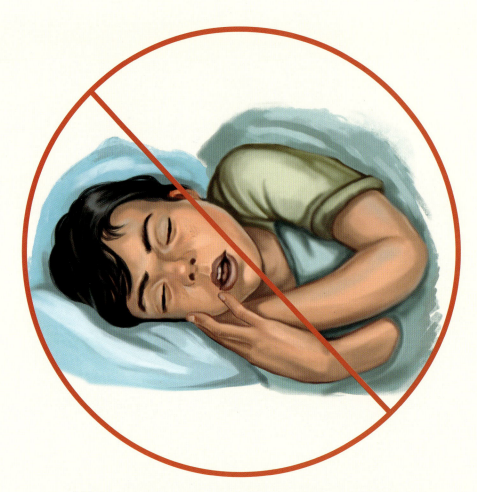

When sleeping open mouthed, expect problems!

(You will snore…)

PEOPLE WILL LIKE SPENDING TIME WITH YOU MORE

We all like it when people listen to us. Sometimes it feels like they don't but maybe it's only because they can't understand you. When you speak clearly and stop to let people listen and reply, it's more fun for everyone!

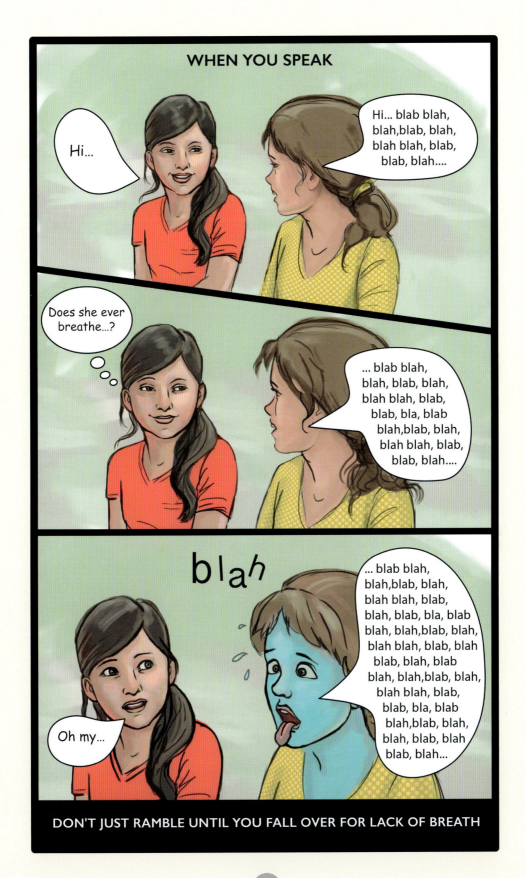

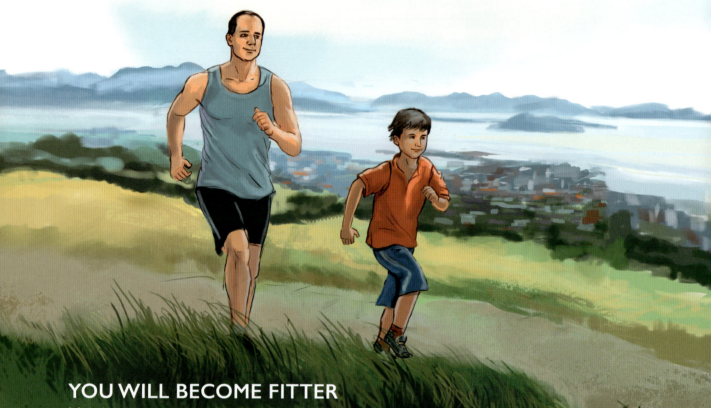

YOU WILL BECOME FITTER

Using your nose to breathe is harder, it makes your body become more efficient with the amount of air it has to use. That is the secret to fitness, learning to do more with less!

Take time each day to play outside or do some exercise and keep your mouth closed as much as you can. You might be surprised if you keep this up, you will notice how much longer it takes before you begin to huff and puff through your mouth!

Start by walking with your mouth closed and only breathe through your nose. See how long you can walk before you need more air and have to use your mouth. This tells you how fit your body is. The longer you can do it, the fitter you are!

Try to leave your mouth closed longer and longer each day you do your walk. Later you might even try to run with your mouth closed. The longer you take to use your mouth to breath, the fitter you become. Don't be surprised if your friends fall behind, be nice and wait for them!

OTHER BENEFITS:

Smarter! Winning is often about being disciplined and working hard, doing the right thing for others and for you.

Happier! You have a powerful secret, one that can change who you are and transform you into the very best you can be. That's the luckiest gift anyone can have!

The fact that you will grow taller, have straighter teeth and look better are just added bonus!

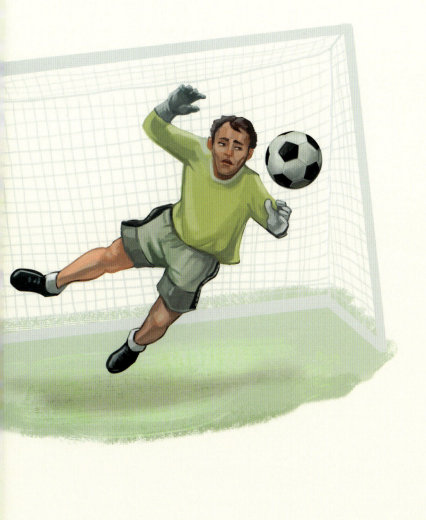
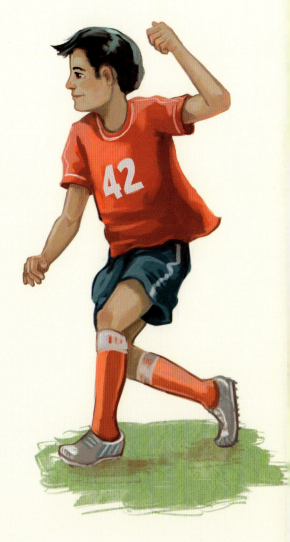

Summing Everest by heli drop is a sure fire way to big achievements. But don't forget, an easy lift up doesn't always provide a safe landing down! Very often, worthy achievements really are just a series of small uphill steps!

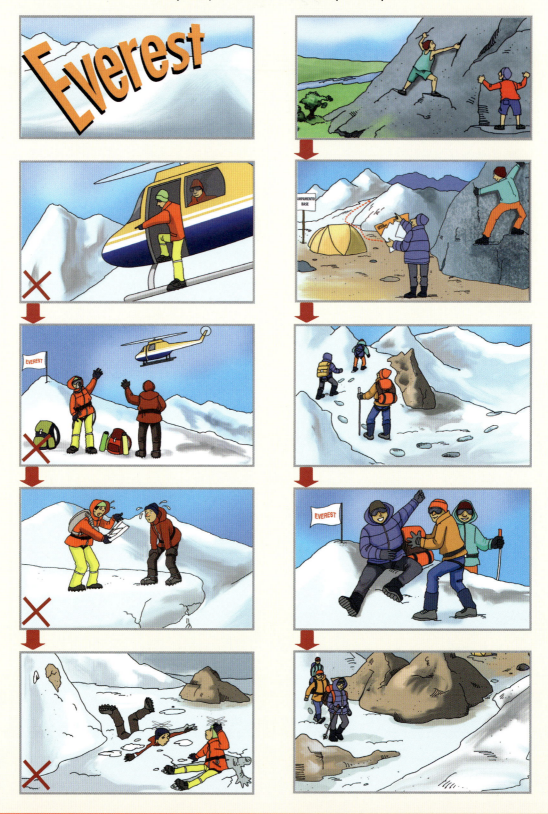

**GOPex IS THE PREPARATION
30 CONSECUTIVE DAYS OF "*SMALL* UPHILL STEPS"**

FOR PARENTS:
GOPex DEMANDS "Constant Dedicated Discipline"

The success or failure of GOPEX during and after the 30-day journey relies 100% on you as parent and the total discipline that YOU must apply. If you are not ready to dedicate everything to change every aspect of your child's behavior then this program is not the right option for you.

This book includes work for your child, yet each of those items requires just as much from you. While these techniques are simple, they are not easy. The tasks have been designed to make them look simple for your children to perform. Mastery of these tasks by your child is not easy and requires you, the parent, to be unwavering in your diligence to insure your child's absolute and strict dedication in the short and long-term.

POSTURE AND FUNCTION

The reason why this system is not even more popular is due to the fact that most dental professionals do not understand the importance of distinguishing oral "posture" from "function".

Function is related to activities such as speaking, chewing and swallowing.

Posture is the mouth's resting state while it is not performing those functional tasks.

The 30-day challenge, properly performed, trains the brain and the body to know how to be in the "correct" resting state (aka: oral posture). The resting state of the tongue significantly impacts facial growth through continuous pressure. We, all of us, spend more time resting than actively performing functional tasks.

As a parent you must be constantly vigilant to promote the right Oral Posture by monitoring your child in their resting state.

DR. WONG SAYS:

"My job is to position your children as close as possible to their peak potential. I am biased: you need to prioritize this over any other activity. Your child's health and wellbeing is my priority. If you feel we are on the same page, I can guide you."

CASE STUDY

Jane and Ally had both struggled with developing the posture changes that the exercises aimed to achieve. They were very consistent with the program but only noticed small improvements in Ally's posture.
Jane made the decision to take some time off from work, pulled Ally out of school to keep her home where she could watch her all the time and track her progress.

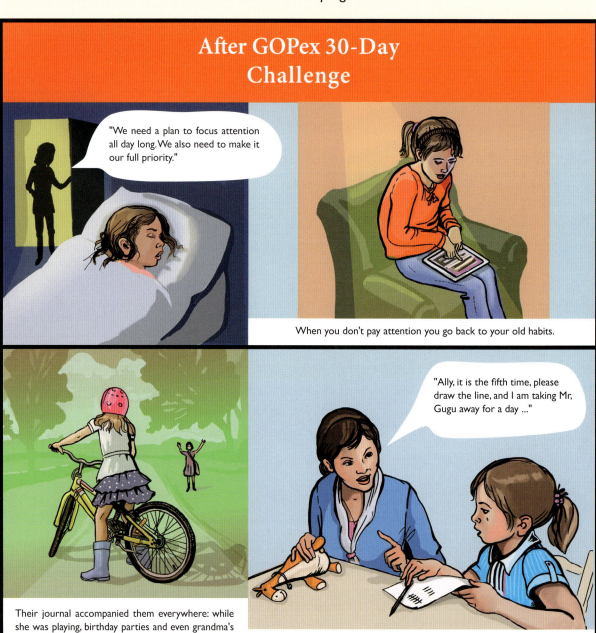

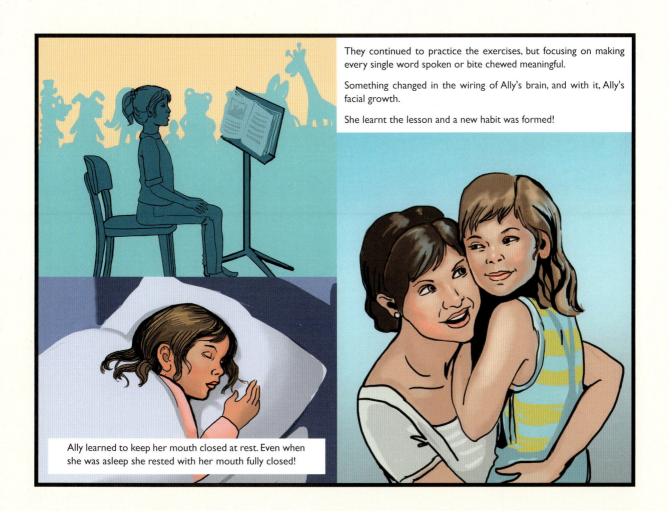

Most parents have a hard time causing distress to their children. However, if a parent really understands the long term health consequences of poor oral posture, they will surely do everything to make sure their children practice GOPex regularly and successfully. After all, what wouldn't you do to watch your child grow healthy, fitter and stronger?

At the end of the day the parents are the ones that can make or break this program!

REMEMBER

The most important thing to remember is that GOPex is a series of very simple exercises. These exercises are not magical, but they are a means to change your habits. They require constant effort to work. They teach and help you keep your mouth fully closed at rest in its proper position.

Use the exercises but most importantly: always remind yourself to keep your mouth closed as we demonstrated.

Undoubtedly, one of the most important decisions you can make for your health is to choose to practice the Exercises of Good Oral Posture - GOPex.

Joaquín Muñoz says:

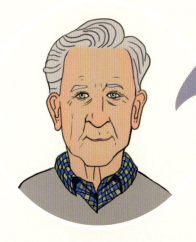

"Good manners and nice posture will open doors for you!"

FINAL WORD

A NOTE TO ALL PARENTS:

We all want to comfort and protect our children. This is our basic survival and human nature. Yet deep within ourselves, we also wish them all their youthful dreams. So let us not hinder them with our own fears but instead prepare them a safe passage in this world by teaching them discipline through hard work!

Visit our website www.forwardontics.com to know more!

100% GOPex

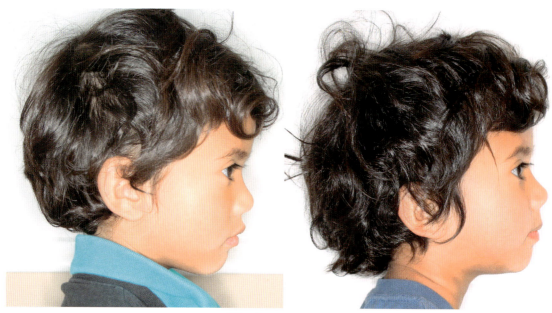

**30 day GOPex
3 years old**

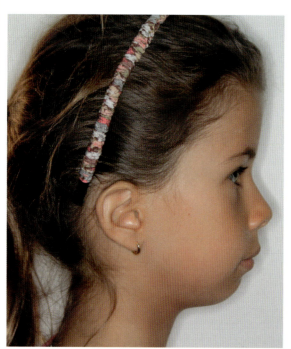 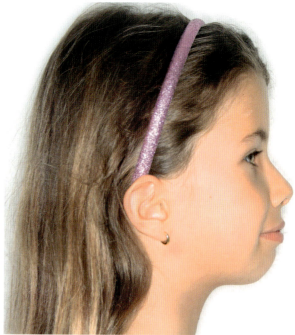

**5 month GOPex
7 years old**

100% GOPex

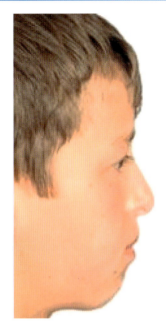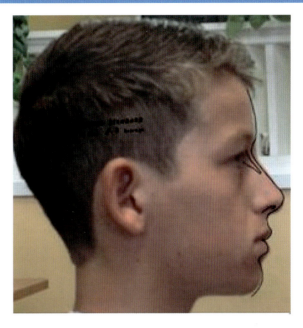

GOPex + Biobloc Orthotropics

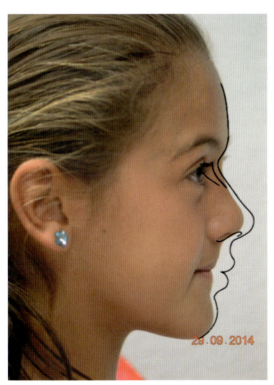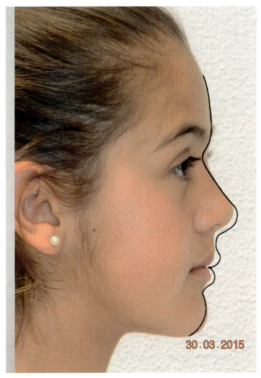

**6 month GOPex
10 years old**

GOPex 30-Day Challange

MONTHLY WORKBOOK FOR _____ **START DAY** _____

EXERCISES	1	2	3	4	5	6	7	8	9	10	11	12	13	14	15	16	17	18	19	20	21	22	23	24	25	26	27	28	29	30
Click'n Close / N position																														
Tongue Push-ups 6 x10 reps																														
Morning Counting 1 min																														
Focused Chewing 2 min x 3																														
Evening Counting 1 min																														
Open Mouth Smiles																														
Reading out Loud 5 -10 min																														
HYGIENE																														
Morning Teeth Brushing																														
Evening Teeth Brushing																														
Weekly Teeth Plaque Disclosure																														
SLEEP																														
Open Mouth / Snoring																														
Grinding																														
ACKNOWLEDGEMENT																														
Love You Hugs Dad 30 sec																														
Love You Hugs Mom 30 sec																														

COMMENTS _____

***Parents please supervise and assist your child (where necessary). Both supervising adult and child are to initial each task each day.*
***Remember to bring your sheets with you to your appointments.*

PHOTOCOPY BEFORE FILLING-IN SO YOU CAN USE IT DURING YOUR WHOLE TREATMENT.